Clinical
Applications
of Human
Anatomy
A Laboratory Guide

Clinical Applications *of* Human Anatomy

A Laboratory Guide

Michael F. Nolan, PhD, PT

Department of Anatomy
University of South Florida
College of Medicine
Tampa, FL

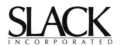

SLACK
INCORPORATED

An innovative information, education, and management company
6900 Grove Road • Thorofare, NJ 08086

The procedures and practices described in this book should be implemented in a manner consistent with the professional standards set for the circumstances that apply in each specific situation. Every effort has been made to confirm the accuracy of the information presented and to correctly relate generally accepted practices. The author, editor, and publisher cannot accept responsibility for errors or exclusions or for the outcome of the application of the material presented herein. There is no expressed or implied warranty of this book or information imparted by it.

Any review or mention of specific companies or products is not intended as an endorsement by the author or publisher.

The work SLACK Incorporated publishes is peer reviewed. Prior to publication, recognized leaders in the field, educators, and clinicians provide important feedback on the concepts and content that we publish. We welcome feedback on this work.

This book has been bound with a revolutionary adhesive process called lay flat binding. Using this binding results in a book with a free-floating cover and a flexible spine, allowing the book to open flat for greater ease of use.

Nolan, Michael F.
Clinical applications of human anatomy: a laboratory guide / Michael F. Nolan.
p. cm.
Includes index.
ISBN 1-55642-598-8
1. Human anatomy--Laboratory manuals. 2. Palpation--Laboratory manuals.
[DNLM: 1. Anatomy--Laboratory Manuals. 2. Anatomy--Problems and Exercises. 3. Auscultation--Laboratory Manuals. 4. Auscultation--Problems and Exercises. 5. Palpation--Laboratory Manuals. 6. Palpation--Problems and Exercises. QS 25 N788c 2003] I. Title.
QM34.N64 2003 611--dc 21
2003001552

Printed in the United States of America.

Published by: SLACK Incorporated
                  6900 Grove Road
                  Thorofare, NJ 08086 USA
                  Telephone: 856-848-1000
                  Fax: 856-853-5991
                  www.slackbooks.com

Contact SLACK Incorporated for more information about other books in this field or about the availability of our books from distributors outside the United States.

For permission to reprint material in another publication, contact SLACK Incorporated. Authorization to photocopy items for internal, personal, or academic use is granted by SLACK Incorporated provided that the appropriate fee is paid directly to Copyright Clearance Center. Prior to photocopying items, please contact the Copyright Clearance Center at 222 Rosewood Drive, Danvers, MA 01923 USA; phone: 978-750-8400; website: www.copyright.com; email: info@copyright.com.

For further information on CCC, check CCC Online at the following address: http://www.copyright.com.

Last digit is print number: 10 9 8 7 6 5 4 3 2 1

DEDICATION

This work is dedicated to my lovely wife and best friend, Debby.

CONTENTS

Section I.   Limbs and Back

Section II.   Thorax and Abdomen

Section III. Head and Neck

ABOUT THE AUTHOR

Dr. Michael F. Nolan received a Bachelor's degree in Physical Therapy from Marquette University and a PhD in Anatomy (Neuroanatomy) from the Medical College of Wisconsin. He holds the rank of Professor in the departments of Anatomy and Neurology in the College of Medicine at the University of South Florida in Tampa.

Dr. Nolan is the director of Applied Neuroscience and Clinical Neuroanatomy courses for medical students, physical therapy students, and neurology and neurosurgery residents at the University of South Florida. He is the author of *Introduction to the Neurologic Examination* and is currently working on a textbook and laboratory guide in the applied neurosciences.

PREFACE

The ability to relieve discomfort and effectively treat injury, disease, and disability requires a clear understanding of the structural and functional bases of a variety of abnormal conditions. Such knowledge of abnormal structure and function is most effectively acquired and easily accessed when it is built upon a firm understanding of normal structure and function. Thus, one of the first goals of students of the health care professions is to acquire an adequate working knowledge of normal structure and function, including variations in structure and ranges in function that are commonly understood to represent the normal condition.

The structure of the human body is usually considered in courses in gross anatomy. These courses typically consist of lectures by the faculty, readings in assigned textbooks, and the study of photographs and illustrations in human anatomy atlases. Depending on the resources of the educational program, students may also have access to skeletal material, anatomical models, videotape presentations of cadaver prosections, and other specialized learning aids. More recently, computer-aided instruction programs have been developed that combine a number of self-directed learning and assessment strategies.

Some gross anatomy courses offer the opportunity to dissect and study human cadaveric material, thereby providing students with a somewhat more realistic, three-dimensional perspective of individual tissues and organs and their anatomical relationship to one another. The use of cadavers and cadaveric material is considered by many to be essential for students requiring a thorough and complete knowledge of human structure.

However, as students progress through the curriculum and move into the more clinical or practice oriented phases, many discover that the anatomical knowledge they actually need is somewhat different from the kind they possess. What many encounter is difficulty in applying the facts and principles previously learned in the classroom and dissection laboratory in the clinical setting. This difficulty often becomes evident in clinical skills courses in which students work with and learn from living persons, many of whom are patients. Student difficulty in making this transition points to a need which can be effectively addressed within the context of most human anatomy courses. Namely, the need to acquire a fundamental understanding of anatomical structure and relationships as encountered in living persons. The practical exercises in this manual are intended to help meet that need.

Michael F. Nolan, PhD, PT

INTRODUCTION

The exercises in this manual are intended to bridge the gap between non-living and living anatomy by helping students acquire a practical understanding of certain aspects of human gross anatomy that can be appreciated in living human subjects. This manual is intended for use as a companion text in conjunction with traditional courses in human gross anatomy, whether or not such courses also provide opportunities to dissect and study cadaveric material. The decision to not include anatomical photographs or illustrations in the manual itself represents a deliberate effort to keep the cost of the book down so that it might be financially within the reach of as many students of human anatomy as possible. Contemporary anatomy texts and atlases (as well as many of the newer sources on the Internet) that students would otherwise be required to purchase in connection with courses in human anatomy are typically well-illustrated and might easily be used should students find the need for such illustrative material.

Individual exercises have been developed with an eye toward preparing students for subsequent course work that may be dependent on a firm understanding of human gross anatomy. The fill-in-the-blank questions are intended for use as a self-assessment tool and to provide feedback with regard to a student's success in learning the material.

An important goal in preparing this manual was to better integrate material that is more often than not treated separately in contemporary health care curricula. It is hoped that through this integration students will more quickly develop an appreciation of the importance and relevance of human anatomy.

How to Use this Manual

The exercises described in this manual are group activities, intended and designed for small numbers of students working together. Each work group should ideally consist of four to six students, preferably mixed with regard to body size, shape, age, gender, and race. The intent of building diversity within the work group is to permit students to gain familiarity with as wide a variety of human anatomy as class enrollment will permit. Students should dress in comfortable clothing that does not prohibit visualization or palpation of important anatomical landmarks and structures.

Each student in the work group should take a turn as the subject for each exercise performed by each of the other members of the group. Clearly, the greatest benefit is achieved when each student performs each exercise on all other members of the group. In this way, variations in anatomical structure that exist within the group can be identified, compared, and discussed in relation to a student's developing concept of normal human anatomy. The short written questions that accompany many of the exercises can be answered as one progresses through the manual as a way of self-assessment and as a prompt for thought and discussion about the anatomy being studied. Alternatively, they can be answered before performing the exercises as a way of preparing for the subsequent group work. Where there is one line following a question, only one answer is sought. Where more than one line is provided, an equivalent number of answers is sought.

Many of the exercises described in this manual involve palpation and learning through the sense of touch. This approach to learning human anatomy, though overlooked in most traditional anatomy courses, is emphasized here in recognition of the fact that physicians and other health care workers regularly use their hands as well as their eyes and ears to obtain information about their patients. It is therefore important for students to become familiar with human structure as it appears to the hands and fingertips. Not coincidentally, many of the exercises and tasks outlined in this manual are similar or identical to those actually used in the evaluation and treatment of patients. Please view these learning activities as serious and necessary parts of your educational and professional development, and treat your work group partners with the respect and sensitivity you would wish them to extend to you.

LIMBS AND BACK

Shoulder Girdle and Upper Limb

INSPECTION AND PALPATION

With the subject seated comfortably and the back, shoulders, and upper limbs exposed:

1. **Inspect and palpate the superior border of the trapezius.**

   a. Are the right and left sides visually symmetrical with regard to muscle contour and bulk? _____

   If not, describe the differences. _____

   _____

   b. Are the right and left sides symmetrical to palpation? _____

   If not, describe the differences. _____

   _____

2. **Inspect and palpate the clavicle from the sternoclavicular joint to the acromioclavicular joint.**

   a. What kind of movement is permitted at the sternoclavicular joint?

   _____

b. What kind of movement is permitted at the acromioclavicular joint?

_____

3. **Inspect the deltoid muscle and palpate the anterior and posterior margins of this muscle.**

   a. Are the right and left sides visually symmetrical with regard to muscle contour and bulk? _____

   If not, describe the differences. _____

   _____

   b. Are the right and left sides symmetrical to palpation? _____

   If not, describe the differences. _____

   _____

4. **Palpate the spine of the scapula from its medial to lateral extent.**

   a. What is the name of the bony prominence at the lateral end of the spine of the scapula? _____

   b. In a relaxed individual with both arms hanging comfortably at the sides, which thoracic vertebral body would be crossed by a line interconnecting the medial edge of the spines of the two scapulae? _____

   c. Which muscle originates in the space superior to the spine of the scapula?

   _____

      1. Which peripheral nerve provides motor innervation to this muscle?

   _____

   d. Which muscle originates in the space inferior to the spine of the scapula?

   _____

1. Which peripheral nerve provides motor innervation to this muscle?

_____

5. **Palpate the vertebral border, lateral border, and inferior angle of the scapula.**

    a. What is the average distance between the spinous processes of the vertebral column and the vertebral border of the scapula? _____

    b. Which rib is covered by the superior angle of the scapula? _____

    c. Which rib is covered by the inferior angle of the scapula?_____

6. **Palpate the anterior and posterior axillary folds.**

    a. Which muscle forms the anterior axillary fold? _____

       1. Which two peripheral nerves provide motor innervation to this muscle?

       _____

       _____

    b. Which two muscles form the posterior axillary fold?

       _____

       _____

       1. Which two peripheral nerves provide motor innervation to these muscles? _____

       _____

7. **Inspect and palpate the muscles of the anterior compartment of the arm.**

    a. Which two muscles form the bulk of the anterior compartment of the arm?

       _____

       _____

1. Which peripheral nerve provides motor innervation to these muscles?

_____

b. Are the right and left sides visually symmetrical with regard to muscle contour and bulk? _____

If not, describe the differences. _____

_____

8. **Inspect and palpate the muscles of the posterior compartment of the arm.**

   a. Which muscle forms the bulk of the posterior compartment of the arm?

   _____

   1. Which peripheral nerve provides motor innervation to this muscle?

   _____

   b. Are the right and left sides visually symmetrical with regard to muscle contour and bulk? _____

   If not, describe the differences. _____

   _____

9. **Inspect and palpate the olecranon process of the ulna.**

   a. Which muscle inserts on the olecranon process? _____

   b. Which peripheral nerve lies immediately medial to the olecranon process?

   _____

10. **Inspect and palpate the medial supracondylar ridge and medial epicondyle of the humerus.**

a. What are the three major actions of the muscles that originate from the medial supracondylar ridge and medial epicondyle?

1. _____

2. _____

3. _____

11. **Inspect and palpate the lateral supracondylar ridge and lateral epicondyle of the humerus.**

a. What are the three major actions of the muscles that originate from the lateral supracondylar ridge and lateral epicondyle?

1. _____

2. _____

3. _____

12. **Inspect and palpate the medial and lateral margins of the antecubital fossa.**

a. Which muscle forms the inferomedial border of the antecubital fossa?

_____

1. Which peripheral nerve provides motor innervation to this muscle?

_____

b. Which muscle forms the inferolateral border of the antecubital fossa?

_____

1. Which peripheral nerve provides motor innervation to this muscle?

_____

c. Which artery lies on the floor of the antecubital fossa? _____

d. Which vein lies superficial in the antecubital fossa? _____

   e. The median nerve enters the forearm from the antecubital fossa by passing between the two heads of origin of the _____

   f. The ulnar nerve enters the forearm from behind the medial epicondyle of the humerus by passing between the two heads of origin of the

_____

13. **Inspect and palpate the muscles of the posterior compartment of the forearm.**

   a. Are the right and left sides visually symmetrical with regard to muscle bulk and contour? _____

   b. Are the right and left sides symmetrical to palpation? _____

     If not, describe the differences. _____

_____

   c. Which peripheral nerve provides motor innervation to these muscles?

_____

14. **Inspect and palpate the muscles of the anterior compartment of the forearm.**

   a. Are the right and left sides visually symmetrical with regard to muscle bulk and contour? _____

   b. Are the right and left sides symmetrical to palpation? _____

     If not, describe the differences. _____

_____

   c. Which two peripheral nerves provide motor innervation to these muscles?

_____

_____

15. **Palpate each of the following:**

    a. Head of the ulna

    b. Pisiform bone

    c. Styloid process of the radius

    d. Dorsal (Lister's) tubercle of the radius

        1. Which tendon lies along the ulnar side of Lister's tubercle?

        _____

16. **At the level of the proximal wrist crease, identify and palpate the tendons of the:**

    a. Flexor carpi radialis

    b. Palmaris longus

    c. Flexor carpi ulnaris

    d. Which artery lies on the radial side of the tendon of the flexor carpi radialis?

        _____

    e. Which artery lies on the radial side of the tendon of the flexor carpi ulnaris?

        _____

    f. Which nerve lies on the radial side of the tendon of the palmaris longus?

        _____

17. **Identify and inspect the transverse and longitudinal flexion creases of the palm.**

18. **Inspect and palpate the thenar and hypothenar eminences.**

    a. Are the right and left sides visually symmetrical with regard to muscle bulk and contour? _____

    If not, describe the differences. _____

    _____

    b. Which three muscles form the bulk of the thenar eminence?

       1. _____

       2. _____

       3. _____

    c. Which peripheral nerve provides motor innervation to these muscles?

       _____

    d. Which three muscles form the bulk of the hypothenar eminence?

       1. _____

       2. _____

       3. _____

    e. Which peripheral nerve provides motor innervation to these muscles?

       _____

19. **Identify and palpate the medial and lateral margins of the anatomical snuff box.**

    a. Which muscle forms the medial (ulnar) border of the anatomical snuff box?

       _____

b. Which two muscles form the lateral (radial) border of the anatomical snuff box?

1. _____

2. _____

c. Which artery lies on the floor of the anatomical snuff box? _____

20. Inspect and palpate the bellies of the dorsal interossei between adjacent metacarpal bones.

a. Are the right and left sides visually symmetrical with regard to muscle bulk?

_____

If not, describe the differences. _____

_____

b. What is the action of the dorsal interossei? _____

c. Which nerve innervates the dorsal interossei? _____

d. What is the action of the palmar interossei? _____

e. Which nerve innervates the palmar interossei? _____

MOVEMENT (MUSCLES AND JOINTS)

Instruct the subject to perform each of the following movements and to maintain the new position while you attempt to move the body part to the starting position. Examine the strength of both the right and left sides. Note the full range of motion permitted at each joint and the strength needed by the subject to resist your efforts to reposition the body part. In the spaces provided, list the main muscles responsible for each movement and indicate the peripheral nerve that innervates each muscle. With the subject in the sitting position, ask the subject to:

Muscle   *Nerve*

1. Elevate (shrug) the shoulders.

    a. _____   _____

    b. _____   _____

2. Retract the shoulders (adduct the scapulae).

    a. _____   _____

    b. _____   _____

    c. _____   _____

3. Flex the arm through the full range of motion.

    a. _____   _____

Muscle   *Nerve*

4. **Abduct the arm through the full range of motion.**

     a. _____   _____

     b. _____   _____

5. **Adduct the abducted arm.**

     a. _____   _____

     b. _____   _____

     c. _____   _____

     d. _____   _____

6. **Hyperextend the arm through the full range of motion.**

     a. _____   _____

     b. _____   _____

7. **Flex the forearm (elbow) with the forearm supinated.**

     a. _____   _____

     b. _____   _____

Muscle   **Nerve**

8. **Flex the forearm (elbow) with the forearm pronated.**

     a. _____   _____

     b. _____   _____

9. **Extend the forearm (elbow) from the fully flexed position.**

     a. _____   _____

10. **Pronate the supinated forearm.**

     a. _____   _____

     b. _____   _____

11. **Supinate the pronated forearm.**

     a. _____   _____

     b. _____   _____

12. **Extend the wrist.**

     a. _____   _____

     b. _____   _____

     c. _____   _____

Muscle   **Nerve**

13. **Flex the wrist.**

    a. _____   _____

    b. _____   _____

14. **Deviate the wrist in a radial direction.**

    a. _____   _____

    b. _____   _____

    c. _____   _____

15. **Deviate the wrist in an ulnar direction.**

    a. _____   _____

    b. _____   _____

16. **Abduct the thumb.**

    a. _____   _____

    b. _____   _____

Muscle   **Nerve**

17. Adduct the thumb.

a. _____   _____

18. Flex the thumb.

a. _____   _____

b. _____   _____

19. Extend the thumb.

a. _____   _____

b. _____   _____

c. _____   _____

20. Oppose the thumb and little finger.

a. _____   _____

b. _____   _____

21. Flex the metacarpophalangeal joints of the medial four fingers.

a. _____   _____

Muscle   Nerve

22. **Extend the metacarpophalangeal joints of the medial four fingers.**

    a. _____   _____

23. **Abduct the fingers.**

    a. _____   _____

24. **Adduct the fingers.**

    a. _____   _____

25. **Flex the fingers at the proximal interphalangeal (PIP) joints.**

    a. _____   _____

26. **Flex the fingers at the distal interphalangeal (DIP) joints.**

    a. _____   _____

27. **Extend the fingers at the PIP and DIP joints.**

    a. _____   _____

VASCULATURE (VEINS AND ARTERIES)

1. **With the aid of an elastic tourniquet wrapped around the arm near the axilla, identify the following superficial veins throughout their course:**

   a. Basilic vein

   b. Cephalic vein

   c. Median cubital vein

   d. Median antecubital vein

2. **Locate and palpate the following arterial pulses:**

   a. Brachial artery in the arm

   b. Brachial artery in the antecubital fossa

   c. Radial artery at the wrist

   d. Ulnar artery at the wrist

   e. Radial artery in the anatomical snuff box

PERIPHERAL NERVES

1. **On the right upper limb of a subject, outline the area of skin innervated by nerve fibers comprising each of the following spinal dorsal roots:**

   a. C5

   b. C6

   c. C7

   d. C8

   e. T1

2. **An autonomous zone is an area of skin generally understood to be innervated exclusively by afferent (sensory) nerve fibers contained within a single pre-plexus spinal nerve root or post-plexus peripheral nerve. On the right upper limb, identify and mark the autonomous zone for each of the following spinal dorsal roots:**

   a. C5

   b. C6

c. C7

d. C8

e. T1

3. **On the left upper limb of the same subject, outline the area of skin inner-vated by nerve fibers comprising each of the following peripheral nerves:**

   a. Upper lateral brachial cutaneous nerve

   b. Lower lateral brachial cutaneous nerve

   c. Posterior brachial cutaneous nerve

   d. Medial brachial cutaneous nerve

   e. Lateral antebrachial cutaneous nerve

   f. Posterior antebrachial cutaneous nerve

   g. Medial antebrachial cutaneous nerve

   h. Median nerve in the hand

   i. Ulnar nerve in the hand

   j. Radial nerve in the hand

4. **On the left upper limb, identify and mark the autonomous zone for each of the following peripheral nerves:**

   a. Axillary nerve

   b. Lateral antebrachial cutaneous nerve

   c. Deep radial nerve

   d. Median nerve

   e. Ulnar nerve

   f. Medial antebrachial cutaneous nerve

   g. Medial brachial cutaneous nerve

5. **The brachial plexus passes from the root of the neck into the axilla by cours-ing over the top of the first rib between two muscles. These two muscles are:**

   a. _____

   b. _____

Hip Girdle
and Lower Limb

INSPECTION AND PALPATION

With the subject resting comfortably in the supine position, perform the following:

1. **Identify and palpate the greater trochanter.**

2. **Identify the location of the inguinal ligament by placing the tip of your long finger on the pubic tubercle and the tip of your thumb on the anterior superior iliac spine. (Note: use your right hand when identifying the subject's right inguinal ligament and your left hand when identifying the left inguinal ligament.)**

   a. Which artery courses deep to the inguinal ligament midway between the anterior superior iliac spine and the pubic tubercle? _____

   b. Which structure lies medial to the artery beneath the inguinal ligament?

   _____

c. Which structure lies lateral to the artery beneath the inguinal ligament?

_____

d. Which muscles form the borders of the femoral triangle?

1. _____

2. _____

3. **Inspect and palpate the quadriceps femoris muscle. Pay particular attention to the distally located oblique fibers of the vastus medialis (VMO).**

a. Are the right and left sides visually symmetrical with regard to muscle contour and bulk? _____

If not, describe the differences. _____

_____

b. Which of the four heads of this muscle does NOT originate from the femur?

_____

c. What is the origin of this part of the quadriceps femoris?

_____

4. **Instruct the subject to contract the quadriceps (forcefully extend the knee) while you palpate the distal part of the vastus medialis.**

a. Are the two sides symmetrical to palpation? _____

If not, describe the differences. _____

_____

b. What effect does the action of this part of the quadriceps have on the patella?

_____

5. **Inspect and palpate the patellar ligament.**

    a. What is the proximal attachment of this ligament? _____

    b. What is the distal attachment of this ligament? _____

6. **Inspect and palpate the fibular head.**

    a. Which nerve lies along the posterior surface of the fibular head? _____

    _____

    b. Which muscle originates on the fibular head? _____

7. **Inspect and palpate the tibial tubercle and anterior tibial crest.**

    a. What are the major actions of the muscles in the anterior compartment of the leg?

    1. _____

    2. _____

    b. Which peripheral nerve lies within the anterior compartment of the leg?

    _____

    c. Which artery lies in the anterior compartment of the leg? _____

    _____

8. **Inspect and palpate the lateral malleolus and medial malleolus.**

    a. Which two muscles have tendons that lie posterior to the lateral malleolus?

    1. _____

    2. _____

9. **Inspect the medial and lateral longitudinal arches of the foot.**

   a. What is the most important ligament supporting the medial longitudinal arch? _____

10. **Inspect the toes.**

    a. Does the subject have hallux valgus? _____

    b. Does the subject have hammer toes? _____

With the subject lying comfortably in the supine position, slide one foot toward the buttock until the knee is flexed 90 degrees. Keep the foot flat on the examination table.

11. **Grasp the leg with both hands just below the knee and gently pull the tibia away from the buttock while keeping the foot immobile.**

    a. Which ligament prevents anterior displacement of the tibia on the femur?

    _____

    b. What is the tibial attachment of this ligament? _____

    c. What is the femoral attachment of this ligament? _____

12. **Grasp the leg with both hands just below the knee and gently push the tibia toward the buttock while keeping the foot immobile.**

    a. Which ligament prevents posterior displacement of the tibia on the femur?

    _____

    b. What is the tibial attachment of this ligament? _____

    c. What is the femoral attachment of this ligament? _____

With the subject lying comfortably in the prone position, perform the following:

13. Palpate the iliac crests.

a. Which vertebra would be crossed by a line interconnecting the superior margins of the iliac crests? _____

14. Palpate the ischial tuberosity.

a. Which ligament attaches to the ischial tuberosity? _____

b. Which muscles originate from the ischial tuberosity?

1. _____

2. _____

3. _____

4. _____

15. Inspect and palpate the posterior thigh (hamstring) muscles.

a. Are the right and left sides visually symmetrical with regard to bulk and contour? _____

If not, describe the differences. _____

_____

b. What is the major action of the posterior muscles of the thigh?

_____

16. Inspect and palpate the popliteal fossa.

a. Which muscle forms the superolateral border of the popliteal fossa?

_____

      1. Which two peripheral nerves provide motor innervation to this muscle?

_____

_____

  b. Which two muscles form the superomedial border of the popliteal fossa?

_____

_____

      1. Which peripheral nerve provides motor innervation to these muscles?

_____

  c. Which muscle forms the inferomedial and inferolateral border of the popliteal fossa? _____

      1. Which peripheral nerve provides motor innervation to this muscle?

_____

  d. Which artery lies on the floor of the popliteal fossa? _____

  e. Which nerve lies in the popliteal fossa?_____

  f. Which muscle forms the floor of the popliteal fossa? _____

17. Inspect and palpate the posterior leg (crural) muscles.

  a. Are the right and left sides visually symmetrical with regard to bulk and contour? _____

If not, describe the differences. _____

_____

b. What are the major actions of the muscles of the posterior compartment of the leg?

1. _____

2. _____

c. Which three muscles have tendons that lie posterior to the medial malleolus?

1. _____

2. _____

3. _____

With the subject standing with the feet approximately 6-8 inches apart and the toes parallel and directed forward:

18. Inspect the medial longitudinal arch of the foot.

a. Are the right and left arches symmetrical with regard to the height of the arch? _____

If not, describe the differences. _____

_____

b. Which muscle of the leg helps support the medial longitudinal arch of the foot? _____

MOVEMENT (MUSCLES AND JOINTS)

Instruct the subject to perform each of the following movements and to maintain the new position while you attempt to move the body part to the starting position. Examine movement and strength on both the right and left side. Note the full range of motion permitted at each joint and the strength needed by the subject to resist your efforts to reposition the body part. In the spaces provided, list the main muscles responsible for each movement and indicate the peripheral nerve that innervates each muscle.

With the subject in the sitting position, instruct the subject to:

Muscle　　　　　　　**Nerve**

1. Flex the thigh (hip joint).

　　a. _____　　_____

　　b. _____　　_____

　　c. _____　　_____

2. Extend the leg (knee joint).

　　a. _____　　_____

3. Dorsiflex the foot (ankle joint).

　　a. _____　　_____

4. Plantar flex the foot (ankle joint).

　　a. _____　　_____

　　b. _____　　_____

　　c. _____　　_____

Muscle   Nerve

5. **Extend the toes.**

    a. _____   _____

    b. _____   _____

    c. _____   _____

6. **Flex the toes.**

    a. _____   _____

    b. _____   _____

With the subject lying in the prone position, instruct the subject to:

7. **Hyperextend the thigh (hip joint).**

    a. _____   _____

8. **Flex the leg (knee joint).**

    a. _____   _____

    b. _____   _____

    c. _____   _____

Muscle   *Nerve*

With the subject lying in the supine position, instruct the subject to:

9. Adduct the abducted thigh (hip joint).

    a. _____   _____

    b. _____   _____

    c. _____   _____

10. Abduct the thigh (hip joint).

    a. _____   _____

    b. _____   _____

VASCULATURE (VEINS AND ARTERIES)

1. Palpate the following arterial pulses:

    a. Femoral artery at the level of the inguinal ligament

    b. Popliteal artery

    c. Anterior tibial artery at the ankle

    d. Posterior tibial artery at the talus

    e. Dorsal pedis artery in the foot

NERVES

1. On the right lower limb of a subject, outline the area of skin innervated by sensory nerve fibers comprising each of the following spinal dorsal roots:

    a. L2

    b. L3

    c. L4

    d. L5

    e. S1

    f. S2

2. **On the right lower limb, identify and mark the autonomous zone for each of the following spinal dorsal roots:**

    a. L2

    b. L3

    c. L4

    d. L5

    e. S1

3. **On the left lower limb of the same subject, outline the area of skin innervated by sensory nerve fibers comprising each of the following peripheral nerves:**

    a. Lateral femoral cutaneous nerve

    b. Obturator nerve

    c. Saphenous nerve

    d. Superficial peroneal nerve

    e. Sural nerve

    f. Deep peroneal nerve

4. **On the left lower limb, identify and mark the autonomous zone for each of the following peripheral nerves:**

    a. Lateral femoral cutaneous nerve

    b. Obturator nerve

    c. Saphenous nerve

    d. Superficial peroneal nerve

    e. Sural nerve

    f. Deep peroneal nerve

Back

INSPECTION AND PALPATION

With the subject seated comfortably and the back and shoulders exposed:

1. Inspect the midline of the back from the skull to the sacrum.

   a. Is the vertebral column straight or are there curvatures in either the frontal (coronal) or sagittal plane? _____

   b. Which segments of the vertebral column are concave posteriorly?

   1. _____

   2. _____

   c. An increase in the curvature of either of these parts of the vertebral column in the sagittal plane is referred to as _____

   d. Which segments of the vertebral column are convex posteriorly?

   1. _____

   2. _____

e. An increase in the curvature of the thoracic spine in the sagittal plane is referred to as _____

f. An increase in the curvature of the vertebral column in the coronal plane is referred to as _____

MOVEMENT (MUSCLES AND JOINTS)

The vertebral column is stabilized and intervertebral movement is limited (restricted) by ligaments that interconnect the vertebrae. Name the ligaments that course from:

1. **Vertebral body to vertebral body anteriorly**

    _____

2. **Vertebral body to vertebral body posteriorly**

    _____

3. **Lamina to lamina**

    _____

4. **Transverse process to transverse process**

    _____

5. **Spinous process to spinous process**

    _____

6. **Tip of the spinous process to tip of the spinous process**

    _____

The muscles of the back can be conveniently divided into two groups: the superficially located erector spinae and the more deeply located transversospinal group.

7. **Which muscles comprise the erector spinae?**

    a. _____

    b. _____

    c. _____

8. **Which muscles comprise the transversospinal group?**

    a. _____

    b. _____

    c. _____

9. **The most superficial back muscles in the region of the cervical spine are the:**

    a. _____

    b. _____

10. **The suboccipital muscles play a role in both stabilizing and moving the head on the spine. The major suboccipital muscles are the:**

    a. _____

    b. _____

    c. _____

    d. _____

THORAX AND ABDOMEN

Thorax

INSPECTION AND PALPATION

With the subject seated comfortably facing toward you:

1. **Inspect the sternum**

   a. Is the body of the sternum flat or is it indented (pectus excavatum) or protruded (pectus carinatum)? _____

2. **Palpate the suprasternal (jugular) notch and the sternoclavicular joints.**

   a. Which vertebral body would be crossed by a horizontal line extending posteriorly from the suprasternal notch?_____

3. **Palpate the sternomanubrial joint (sternal angle or angle of Louis).**

   a. Which vertebral body would be crossed by a horizontal line extending posteriorly from the sternomanubrial joint? _____

   b. Which rib attaches to the sternum at the sternal angle? _____

4. **Palpate xiphoid process and xiphisternal joint.**

   a. Which vertebral body would be crossed by a horizontal line extending posteriorly from the xiphisternal joint? _____

   b. Which ribs attach to the sternum by way of their own, individual costal cartilage (ie, vertebrosternal ribs)? _____

   c. Which ribs attach to the sternum by way of a common costal cartilage (ie, vertebrochondral ribs)?_____

5. **Palpate the inferior margin of the costal cartilages starting at the xiphoid process and moving laterally.**

   a. Which ribs attach only to the vertebral column (ie, vertebral ribs)?

   _____

With the subject seated comfortably facing away from you:

6. **Inspect the vertebral column with respect to its position in the sagittal plane.**

   a. Is the convexity of the thoracic spine directed anteriorly or posteriorly?

   _____

   b. What term is used to refer to an increase in the curvature of the thoracic spine in the sagittal plane? _____

7. **Inspect the vertebral column with respect to its position in the coronal plane.**

   a. Is the thoracic spine straight or do you see a curvature?

   _____

   b. If you see a curvature, is the convexity directed toward the right or left side?

   _____

   c. Is the lumbar spine straight or do you see a curvature?

   _____

    d. If you see a curvature, is the convexity directed toward the right or left side?

        _____

    e. What term is used to refer to curvature of the spine in the coronal plane?

        _____

8. **Palpate the spinous process of C7 (vertebra prominens).**
   (Note: Sometimes the spinous process of T1 is prominent to palpation also.)

9. **Palpate the supraspinous ligament from C7 to the sacrum, pressing hard enough to identify the thoracic and lumbar spinous processes.**

10. **With the subject sitting upright and the hands resting lightly on the thighs, palpate the vertebral border of the scapula from the superior angle to the inferior angle.**

    a. Which rib lies immediately deep to the superior angle of the scapula?

        _____

    b. Which rib lies immediately deep to the inferior angle of the scapula?

        _____

LANDMARKS

1. The locations of clinically important structures within the thorax are frequently described in relation to several vertical "lines" that subdivide the thoracic wall into definable regions. With the subject sitting upright and comfortable, identify and mark the following "lines" on the thorax:

   a. Midsternal line

   b. Midclavicular line

   c. Anterior axillary line

   d. Midaxillary line

   e. Posterior axillary line

   f. Midscapular line

   g. Midspinal line

2. Indicate the fiber direction of the external intercostal muscle in the 5th intercostal space on the right side in the anterior axillary line.

3. Indicate the fiber direction of the internal intercostal muscle in the 5th intercostal space on the left side in the anterior axillary line.

4. Which spinal (segmental) nerve provides sensory innervation to the skin of the nipple and areola? _____

Lungs and Pleura

INSPECTION AND PALPATION

With the subject sitting comfortably with the hands resting lightly on the thighs:

1. **Observe the movements of the chest during** *quiet breathing.*

   a. Which phase of the respiratory cycle is longer during quiet breathing?

   _____

   b. What is the normal respiration rate?

   _____

2. **Place the palm and fingers of one hand over the subject's xiphoid process and the other hand over the spinous processes of the T8-T10 vertebrae. Note the extent of chest expansion in the** *anterior-posterior* **direction during quiet breathing. Ask the subject to inhale deeply and exhale fully several times slowly and again note the extent of chest expansion in the** *anterior-posterior* **direction.**

3. Place your hands over the 8th-10th ribs bilaterally in the midaxillary line. Note the extent of chest expansion in the *transverse* direction during quiet breathing. Ask the subject to inhale deeply and exhale fully several times slowly and again note the extent of chest expansion in the *transverse* direction.

LANDMARKS

With the subject sitting comfortably:

1. Identify and mark the pleural reflections on the right and left sides of the thorax.

2. Indicate the rib overlying the pleural reflection in the:
   a. Midclavicular line: _____

   b. Midaxillary line: _____

   c. Midscapular line: _____

3. Which costal cartilage marks the point where the pleural reflection moves laterally beneath the body of the sternum on the *right* side?

   _____

4. Which costal cartilage marks the point where the pleural reflection moves laterally beneath the body of the sternum on the *left* side?

   _____

5. Identify and mark the boundaries of the lungs on the right and left sides.

6. **Which rib overlies the lung boundary in the:**

    a. Midclavicular line: _____

    b. Midaxillary line: _____

    c. Midscapular line: _____

7. **Which costal cartilage marks the point where the medial edge of the *right* lung moves laterally beneath the body of the sternum?**

    _____

8. **Which costal cartilage marks the point where the medial edge of the *left* lung moves laterally beneath the body of the sternum?**

    _____

9. **Identify and mark the location of the oblique fissure of the right and left lungs.**

10. **The oblique fissure lies parallel to a line interconnecting the:**

    a. _____   spinous process posteriorly

    b. _____   rib in the midaxillary line

    c. _____   costal cartilage anteriorly

11. **Identify and mark the location of the horizontal fissure of the right lung.**

12. **The horizontal fissure lies parallel to a line interconnecting the:**

a. _____   in the midaxillary line laterally

b. _____   costal cartilage anteriorly

13. **Name the bronchopulmonary segments of each lung.**

a. Right lung

   1. Superior lobe: _____

                              _____

                              _____

   2. Middle lobe: _____

                              _____

   3. Inferior lobe: _____

                              _____

                              _____

                              _____

b. Left lung

   1. Superior lobe: _____

                              _____

                              _____

                              _____

   2. Inferior lobe: _____

                              _____

                              _____

                              _____

                              _____

14. **The bifurcation of the trachea lies at a level marked by a horizontal line that passes through the:**

    a. _____   anteriorly

    b. _____   posteriorly

15. **Because of its more vertical orientation and slightly greater diameter, an object aspirated into the trachea is more likely to pass into the _____ main stem bronchus.**

16. **Indicate the muscles that form the boundaries of the triangle of auscultation.**

    a. Superomedial boundary: _____

    b. Superolateral boundary: _____

    c. Inferior boundary: _____

17. **Which intercostal space forms the floor of the triangle of auscultation?**

    _____

18. **Name the vertebra that marks the level of the:**

    a. Vena caval foramen: _____

    b. Esophageal hiatus: _____

    c. Aortic hiatus: _____

19. **List the structure that passes through the vena caval foramen.**

    a. _____

20. **List the structures that pass through the esophageal hiatus.**

    a. _____

    b. _____

21. **List the structures that pass through the aortic hiatus.**

    a. _____

    b. _____

    c. _____

Heart

LANDMARKS

With the subject sitting comfortably facing you:

1. **Identify and mark the borders of the heart on the anterior thorax.**

   a. Superior border: Draw a line from the inferior margin of the 2nd costal cartilage on the left to the inferior margin of the 2nd costal cartilage on the right. The line should extend from the left sternal border to the right sternal border.

   b. Right border: Draw a line from the 2nd costal cartilage on the right to the 6th costal cartilage on the right. The line should have a slight convexity toward the right as it courses inferiorly, approximately 1 cm lateral to the lateral sternal border.

   c. Inferior border: Draw a line from the 6th costal cartilage on the right side beginning at the lateral sternal border to the 5th intercostal space on the left side in the midclavicular line.

   d. Left border: Draw a line from the 5th intercostal space on the left side in the midclavicular line to the 2nd costal cartilage on the left along the lateral sternal border.

2. **Identify and mark the anatomical location of the valves of the heart.**

   a. Pulmonary valve: lies posterior to the 3rd sternochondral junction on the left side.

   b. Aortic valve: lies in the midsternal line at the level of the 3rd intercostal space.

   c. Mitral valve: lies posterior to the 4th sternochondral junction on the left side.

   d. Tricuspid valve: lies in the midsternal line at the level of the 5th sternochondral junction.

3. **Identify and mark on the anterior chest wall, sites for auscultating each of the cardiac valves.**

   a. Aortic valve: 2nd intercostal space on the right side along the lateral sternal border.

   b. Pulmonary valve: 2nd intercostal space on the left side along the lateral sternal border.

   c. Tricuspid valve: 5th intercostal space on the left side along the lateral sternal border.

   d. Mitral valve: 5th intercostal space on the left side on or near the midclavicular line.

INSPECTION AND PALPATION

With the subject lying comfortably in the supine position with the head and upper thorax slightly elevated:

1. **Observe the apical impulse.**

   a. Describe the location of the apical impulse.

   _____

2. **While standing on the subject's right side, use your right hand to palpate the point of maximum impulse (PMI).**

   a. Describe the location of the PMI. _____

   _____

   b. What is the subject's heart rate? _____

AUSCULTATION

The cardiac cycle consists of two phases: systole and diastole. During systole the left and right ventricles contract, ejecting blood into the aorta and pulmonary artery, respectively. The onset of systole is marked by closure of the mitral and tricuspid valves (atrioventricular valves). Closure of these valves prevents reflux into the atria and gives rise to the first heart sound (S1). The end of systole (or beginning of diastole) is marked by closure of the aortic and pulmonary valves (semilunar valves). Closure of these valves prevents reflux into the left and right ventricles respectively and gives rise to the second heart sound (S2).

With the subject lying comfortably in the supine position with the head and upper thorax slightly elevated:

1. **Use your stethoscope to auscultate each of the heart valves individually. Which heart sound is loudest or most clearly heard over each valve projection area?**

   a. Aortic area: _____

   b. Tricuspid area: _____

   c. Pulmonary area: _____

   d. Mitral area: _____

2. **In your resting subject, which phase of the cardiac cycle is shorter?**

   _____

Abdomen

INSPECTION

With the subject lying comfortably in the supine position:

1. Inspect the anterior abdominal wall.

a. Is it flat or distended? _____

b. Are there scars or bruises? _____

If so, describe the location, size, length, direction and apparent age.

_____

_____

_____

c. Are there dilated veins visible? _____

If so, describe their location and orientation. _____

_____

_____

2. **Inspect the umbilicus.**

   a. Is the umbilicus in the midline? _____

   b. Is the umbilicus inverted or everted?_____

3. **Inspect the skin overlying the rectus abdominis muscle. Ask the subject to cross the arms over the chest and attempt to lift the shoulders off the table.**

   a. Can you see the lateral borders of the rectus abdominis? _____

   b. Are the tendinous intersections above or below the umbilicus? _____

PALPATION AND LANDMARKS

1. **Palpate and mark the xiphoid process.**

2. **Palpate the inferior margin of the costal cartilages of ribs 6-10. Begin medially at the xiphoid process and move laterally along the costochondral margin until you feel the anterior end of the 11th rib. Mark this border of the anterior abdominal wall on both sides with a line extending from the xiphoid process to the inferior margin of the 11th rib in the midaxillary line.**

3. **Palpate the iliac crests on both sides. Begin laterally in the midaxillary line and move anteriorly until you reach the anterior superior iliac spine (ASIS). Mark this border of the ilium with a line extending from the iliac crest in the midaxillary line to the anterior superior iliac spine on both sides.**

4. **Palpate the inguinal ligament from its superolateral attachment on the anterior superior iliac spine to its inferomedial attachment on the pubic tubercle. Mark this inferior border of the anterior abdominal wall with a line extending from the ASIS to the pubic tubercle.**

The anterior abdominal wall can be divided into four or nine regions by a series of vertical and horizontal lines that intersect identifiable anatomical landmarks. Anatomical landmarks associated with both systems will be identified below.

THE FOUR REGION SYSTEM

5. **Mark a vertical line from the xiphoid process to the pubic symphysis that passes through the umbilicus.**

6. **Mark a horizontal line that passes through the umbilicus (transumbilical line). These two lines define four quadrants identified as the right upper quadrant (RUQ), left upper quadrant (LUQ), right lower quadrant (RLQ) and left lower quadrant (LLQ).**

   a. In a thin subject, what vertebra would be intersected by a horizontal line that extends posteriorly from the umbilicus? _____

7. **List the organs or other important anatomical structures commonly located in each quadrant.**

   a. RUQ: _____   _____

   _____   _____

   _____   _____

   b. LUQ: _____   _____

   _____   _____

   _____

   c. RLQ: _____   _____

   _____   _____

   _____

   d. LLQ: _____   _____

   _____   _____

The Nine Region System

8. **Mark vertical lines on both sides of the abdomen from the costal cartilage to the inguinal ligament in the midclavicular line.**

9. **Mark a horizontal line that passes between the lowest extent of the costal cartilages on each side (subcostal line).**

   a. Which vertebrae would be intersected by a horizontal line extending posteriorly from the subcostal line?_____

   b. Name the three regions of the anterior abdominal wall that lie above the subcostal line.

      1. _____

      2. _____

      3. _____

10. **Mark a horizontal line that passes between the iliac tubercles (transtubercular line).**

    a. Which vertebrae would be intersected by a horizontal line extending posteriorly from the transtubercular line? _____

    b. Name the three regions of the anterior abdominal wall that lie above the transtubercular line and below the subcostal line.

       1. _____

       2. _____

       3. _____

c. Name the three regions of the anterior abdominal wall that lie below the transtubercular line.

1. _____

2. _____

3. _____

11. **Indicate the vertebral level of each of the following:**

a. Bifurcation of the aorta: _____

b. Pyloric valve of the stomach: _____

c. Formation of the inferior vena cava: _____

d. Origin of the inferior mesenteric artery: _____

e. Origin of the renal arteries: _____

12. **Mark a line from the umbilicus to the right ASIS. McBurney's point lies on this line, two thirds the distance from the umbilicus to the ASIS.**

13. **Which spinal (segmental) nerve provides sensory innervation to the skin of the umbilicus?** _____

14. **On the right side of the anterior abdominal wall, indicate the fiber direction of the external oblique muscle.**

15. **On the left side of the anterior abdominal wall, indicate the fiber direction of the internal oblique muscle.**

AUSCULTATION

With the subject lying comfortably in the supine position:

1. **Use your stethoscope to auscultate each of the four quadrants of the anterior abdominal wall. Listen for approximately 3 minutes in each quadrant.**

   a. Did you hear something in each quadrant? _____

   b. Describe the sounds you heard. _____

   _____

   _____

   _____

HEAD AND NECK

Head and Face

INSPECTION AND PALPATION

With the subject seated comfortably facing you:

1. Inspect the position of the head with respect to the neck.

a. Is the head in the midline? _____

If not, is it tilted forward or backward, to the right or left, or rotated (face turned) to the right or left? _____

Describe. _____

_____

_____

b. Is the head held steady or do you see movement? _____

If you see movement, please describe. _____

_____

_____

2. **Palpate the external occipital protuberance.**

   a. What dural venous sinus lies deep to the external occipital protuberance?

   _____

3. **Palpate each of the following bony landmarks.**

   a. Glabella

   b. Nasion

   c. Zygomatic arch

   d. Mental protuberance and tubercles

   e. Angle of the mandible

   f. Mastoid process

      1. Which cranial nerve exits the skull via the stylomastoid foramen?

      _____

4. **Inspect the skin of the forehead.**

   a. Do you see wrinkles? _____

   If so, on which side or both? _____

   _____

5. **Inspect the eyebrows.**

   a. Are they at the same level? _____

   If not, which side is higher?_____

6. **Inspect and measure the height of both palpebral fissures.**

   a. Are they the same height on both sides? _____

If not:

What is the height on the right side? _____

What is the height on the left side? _____

b. Which muscle elevates the upper eyelid? _____

   1. Which cranial nerve innervates this muscle?_____

c. Does the upper lid on either side cover the pupil? _____

  If so, on which side or both? _____

d. Does the upper lid on either side cover the iris? _____

  If so, on which side or both? _____

e. Does the lower lid on either side cover the iris? _____

  If so, on which side or both? _____

f. Do you see more sclera below the iris on one side or the other? _____

_____

  If so, on which side do you see more sclera? _____

g. Is the edge of the lower lid touching the eye? _____

  If not, is the lower lid everted (ectropion) or inverted (entropion)?

_____

   1. Weakness of which muscle causes ectropion? _____

   2. Which cranial nerve innervates this muscle?_____

h. Inspect the conjunctiva of the lower eyelid. Describe its color.

_____

7. **Inspect the nasolabial fold on each side.**

    a. Are the right and left sides symmetrical with regard to depth and definition?

    _____

    If not, describe the differences. _____

    _____

8. **Inspect the corners of the mouth.**

    a. Are the right and left sides symmetrical? _____

    If not, describe the differences. _____

    _____

9. **Inspect the color of the face.**

    a. Is one side more red (hyperemic) than the other? _____

    If so, which side? _____

MOVEMENT

1. **Place your fingers immediately anterior to the tragus on both sides and palpate the movement of the condyle of the mandible as the subject opens and closes the mouth.**

2. **Ask the subject to alternately clench the teeth and relax the bite while you palpate the temporalis and then masseter muscles.**

    a. Which cranial nerve innervates these muscles? _____

3. **Ask the subject to raise the eyebrows.**

    a. Which muscle is used to raise the eyebrows? _____

    b. Which cranial nerve innervates this muscle? _____

4. **Ask the subject to close both eyes tightly.**

   a. Which muscle is used to close the eyes tightly? _____

   b. Which cranial nerve innervates this muscle? _____

   c. Describe Bell's phenomenon. _____

   _____

   _____

   _____

5. **Ask the subject to smile.**

   a. Which muscle is used to retract the corners of the mouth?_____

   b. Which cranial nerve innervates this muscle?_____

6. **Ask the subject to purse the lips as if to whistle.**

   a. Which muscle is used to purse the lips? _____

   b. Which cranial nerve innervates this muscle? _____

7. **Through which foramen does the facial nerve enter the skull (exit the posterior cranial fossa)?** _____

8. **Through which foramen does the facial nerve exit the skull?**

   _____

9. **What are the five terminal branches of the facial nerve that emerge from the substance of the parotid gland?**

   a. _____

   b. _____

   c. _____

   d. _____

   e. _____

VASCULATURE

1. **Palpate pulsations of the superficial temporal artery immediately anterior to the tragus on each side.**

   a. Is the superficial temporal artery a branch of the internal or external carotid artery? _____

2. **Palpate pulsations of the superficial temporal artery in the temporal fossa between the top of the ear and the lateral margin of the eyebrow.**

3. **Palpate pulsations of the facial artery over the body of the mandible between the angle and the mental tubercle.**

   a. Is the facial artery a branch of the internal or external carotid artery?

   _____

PERIPHERAL NERVES

1. **Which cranial nerve mediates sensation from the:**

   a. Forehead over the eyebrows? _____

b. Skin over the maxilla? _____

c. Skin over the mental tubercle? _____

2. **Which cranial nerve provides parasympathetic innervation to the parotid gland?** _____

   a. What is the location of the postganglionic cell body?

   _____

3. **Which cranial nerve provides parasympathetic innervation to the sub-mandibular and submaxillary glands?** _____

   a. What is the location of the postganglionic body?_____

   _____

4. **Which cranial nerve provides parasympathetic innervation to the lacrimal gland?** _____

   a. What is the location of the postganglionic cell body?

   _____

5. **Which cranial nerve provides motor innervation to the muscles of facial expression?** _____

6. **Which cranial nerve provides motor innervation to the muscles of mastica-tion?** _____

7. **Which cranial nerve provides sensory innervation to the face?** _____

   a. Which branch of this nerve innervates the skin over the eyebrow?

   _____

      1. Which opening in the middle cranial fossa contains the axons of this nerve branch? _____

   b. Which branch of this nerve innervates the skin over the maxilla?

   _____

      1. Which opening in the middle cranial fossa contains the axons of this nerve branch? _____

   c. Which branch of this nerve innervates the skin over the mental protuberance?

   _____

      1. Which opening in the middle cranial fossa contains the axons of this nerve branch? _____

8. **Which foramen transmits the axons of the glossopharyngeal nerve?**

   _____

9. **Which striated (skeletal) muscle is innervated by the glossopharyngeal nerve?** _____

10. **Which special sensory functions are mediated by the glossopharyngeal nerve?**

    a. _____

    b. _____

11. Which foramen transmits the axons of the vagus nerve?

   _____

12. Which striated muscles are innervated by the vagus nerve?

   a. _____

   b. _____

13. What is the effect of the vagus nerve on heart rate? _____

   _____

14. What is the effect of the vagus nerve on gastric and intestinal motility?

   _____

   _____

15. Which special sensory functions are mediated by the vagus nerve?

   a. _____

   b. _____

16. Which two foramina transmit the axons of the spinal accessory nerve?

   a. _____

   b. _____

17. **Which muscles are innervated by the spinal accessory nerve?**

    a. _____

    b. _____

18. **Which foramen transmits the axons of the hypoglossal nerve?**

    _____

19. **Which muscle innervated by the hypoglossal nerve is primarily involved in protrusion of the tongue?** _____

Neck

INSPECTION AND PALPATION

With the subject seated comfortably facing you:

1. **Inspect neck from the mastoid process and body of the mandible above to the clavicle and suprasternal notch below.**

   a. Are the two sides visually symmetrical? _____

   If not, describe. _____

   _____

   b. Do you see any masses, swelling, or pulsations? _____

   If so, describe. _____

   _____

2. **Palpate the anterior edge of the sternocleidomastoid muscle from its superior attachment on the mastoid process to its inferior attachment on the clavicle and manubrium. Identify the anterior triangle of the neck.**

   a. Indicate and mark the three boundaries of the anterior triangle of the neck.

   1. _____

   2. _____

   3. _____

   b. Indicate and mark the three boundaries of the carotid triangle.

   1. _____

   2. _____

   3. _____

   c. Indicate the three boundaries of the submandibular triangle.

   1. _____

   2. _____

   3. _____

   d. Indicate and mark the three boundaries of the muscular triangle.

   1. _____

   2. _____

   3. _____

e. Which muscles are located in the muscular triangle?

1. _____

2. _____

3. _____

With the subject seated comfortably facing away from you:

3. **Palpate the angle of the mandible. Move your fingers anteriorly along the inferior margin of the body of the mandible toward the mental protuberance.**

4. **Slide your fingers inferiorly from the body of the mandible and gently palpate the body and greater horns of the hyoid bone.**

    a. What is the vertebral level of the hyoid bone? _____

    b. Indicate the four suprahyoid muscles.

    1. _____

    2. _____

    3. _____

    4. _____

5. **Slide your fingers inferiorly in the anterior midline below the hyoid bone and gently palpate the thyroid notch, laryngeal prominence, and intervening thyrohyoid membrane.**

    a. What is the vertebral level of the thyroid notch? _____

6. **With your fingers on the laryngeal prominence, ask the subject to swallow.**

   a. In which direction does the thyroid cartilage move? _____

   b. Which muscle abducts the vocal folds? _____

   c. Which nerve provides motor innervation to this muscle? _____

   d. Which two muscles adduct the vocal folds?

      1. _____

      2. _____

   e. Which nerve provides motor innervation to these muscles? _____

   f. Which laryngeal muscle lies on the external surface of the larynx?

      _____

   g. Which nerve provides motor innervation to this muscle? _____

   h. Which nerve provides sensory innervation to the mucosal lining of the internal surface of the larynx? _____

7. **Slide your fingers inferiorly in the anterior midline below the thyroid cartilage and gently palpate the cricoid cartilage and intervening cricothyroid membrane.**

   a. What is the vertebral level of the cricoid cartilage? _____

8. Slide your fingers inferiorly in the anterior midline below the cricoid carti-lage and gently palpate the trachea in the space above the suprasternal (jugu-lar) notch. Can you feel the isthmus of the thyroid gland where it lies over the 2-4 tracheal rings? If not, ask the subject to swallow, causing the trachea and overlying thyroid isthmus to move upward beneath your fingertips.

   a. Indicate the four infrahyoid muscles:

      1. _____

      2. _____

      3. _____

      4. _____

9. Palpate the neck along the anterior margin of the sternocleidomastoid mus-cle from the manubrium to the mastoid process and along the posterior and inferior margins of the mandible from the auricle to the mental protuberance.

   a. Do you feel any swollen lymph nodes? _____

      If so, are they tender to palpation? _____

10. Palpate the external occipital protuberance, then slide your fingers inferior-ly along the ligamentum nuchae toward the vertebra prominens.

   a. Vertebra prominens is in the spinous process of which vertebra?

      _____

11. Palpate the anterior border of the trapezius and the posterior border of the sternocleidomastoid from their superior attachments on the skull to their inferior attachments on the clavicle.

   a. Indicate and mark the three boundaries of the posterior triangle of the neck.

      1. _____

      2. _____

      3. _____

b. Mark the course of the spinal accessory nerve as it courses toward the trapezius across the floor of the posterior triangle.

c. Which four muscles form the floor of the posterior triangle of the neck?

1. _____

2. _____

3. _____

4. _____

d. What is the action of the sternocleidomastoid muscle on the head?

_____

12. **Palpate the neck along the posterior margin of the sternocleidomastoid muscle from clavicle to the occipital bone.**

a. Do you feel any swollen lymph nodes? _____

If so, are they tender to palpation? _____

VASCULATURE

With the subject sitting comfortably facing you:

1. **Palpate pulsations of the common carotid artery in the space between the thyroid cartilage and the sternocleidomastoid muscle.**

a. At what vertebral level does the common carotid artery bifurcate?

_____

2. **Palpate pulsations of the internal carotid artery immediately deep to the angle of the mandible.**

   a. Which nerve lies within the carotid sheath along with the carotid artery?

   _____

   b. What other structure lies within the carotid sheath?

   _____

3. **Palpate pulsations of the common carotid in the space between the cricoid cartilage and the sternocleidomastoid muscle.**

   a. Which bony structure lies immediately posterior to the common carotid artery at this level? _____

   b. What is the heart rate of your subject? _____

Chapter 10

Mouth

INSPECTION AND PALPATION

With the subject seated comfortably facing you:

1. **Instruct the subject to open and close the mouth while you palpate the temporomandibular joints bilaterally.**

   a. Are the two sides symmetrical to palpation? _____

   If not, describe what you feel. _____

   _____

2. **Instruct the subject to clench the teeth together while you palpate the mandible immediately anterior and superior to the angle.**

   a. Which muscle do you feel contract beneath your fingers?_____

   b. Which cranial nerve provides motor innervation to this muscle?_____

3. **Instruct the subject to open the mouth widely. With the aid of a penlight, inspect the position of the uvula.**

   a. Is the uvula resting in the midline? _____

   If not, describe its position. _____

   _____

4. **Inspect the lateral walls of the posterior part of the oropharynx.**

   a. Are palatine tonsils present in the tonsillar fossa? _____

   b. Which cranial nerve provides sensory innervation to the posterior part of the oropharynx?_____

   c. Which muscle forms the anterior pillar of the tonsillar fossa? _____

   d. Which muscle forms the posterior pillar of the tonsillar fossa?_____

5. **Inspect the tongue in the relaxed state lying on the floor of the mouth.**

   a. Are the two sides visually symmetrical with regard to muscle bulk?

   _____

   If not, describe the differences. _____

   _____

MOVEMENTS

1. **With the tongue lying relaxed on the floor of the mouth, instruct the subject to say "AAHH".**

   a. Describe the movement of the uvula._____

   b. Which muscle acts to move the uvula during phonation? _____

   c. Which cranial nerve provides motor innervation to this muscle?_____

2. Instruct the subject to protrude the tongue.

    a. Does the tongue protrude in the midline?_____

       If not, describe the deviation. _____

       _____

    b. Which muscle acts to protrude the tongue? _____

    c. Which cranial nerve provides motor innervation to this muscle?_____

    d. Which cranial nerve provides general sensory (cutaneous) innervation to the anterior part of the tongue? _____

    e. Which cranial nerve provides special sensory (taste) innervation to the anterior part of the tongue?_____

Chapter 11

Eye

INSPECTION

Instruct the subject to look straight ahead and focus on some non-moving object at a distance of 20 feet or more.

1. Inspect the sclera in both eyes.

a. What color is the sclera? _____

b. Are the scleral blood vessels engorged or dilated? _____

2. Inspect the iris in both eyes.

a. What color is the iris? _____

b. Are the irides free of defects? _____

If not, describe the defect._____

_____

c. Are the pupils round in both eyes?_____

If not, describe their shape. _____

_____

d. Are the pupils stable in size or do they fluctuate in diameter? _____

3. **What is the diameter of the *right* pupil?** _____

4. **What is the diameter of the *left* pupil?**_____

a. What word is used to describe pupillary asymmetry of greater than 1 mm?

_____

5. **Using a penlight in a room in which the lights have been dimmed, quickly illuminate the *right* eye, taking care to avoid illuminating the left eye.**

a. What effect did you observe in the illuminated right eye?_____

_____

Repeat the procedure described in number 5 above.

b. What effect did you observe in the non-illuminated left eye? _____

_____

c. What reflex did you observe in the illuminated right eye? _____

_____

d. What reflex did you observe in the non-illuminated left eye? _____

_____

6. **Now, quickly illuminate the *left* eye, taking care to avoid illuminating the right eye.**

   a. What effect did you observe in the illuminated left eye? _____

   _____

   Repeat the procedure described in number 6 above.

   b. What effect did you observe in the non-illuminated right eye?_____

   _____

7. **Inspect the position of the eyes in the orbits.**

   a. Are the visual axes of both eyes parallel? _____

   If not, describe the malalignment. _____

   _____

   b. Malalignment of the visual axes is referred to as: _____

   _____

   c. Are the eyes held steady in the orbits? _____

   If not, describe the movements you see. _____

   _____

   _____

   d. Involuntary, oscillating movements of the eyes is called: _____

Movements

1. Indicate the primary and secondary actions of each of the extraocular muscles (assume the eye to be in the position of primary gaze and that the muscle in question is the only muscle acting on the globe).

Muscle	Primary Action	Secondary Actions	
a. Lateral rectus	_____		
b. Medial rectus	_____		
c. Superior rectus	_____	_____	_____
d. Inferior rectus	_____	_____	_____
e. Superior oblique	_____	_____	_____
f. Inferior oblique	_____	_____	_____

2. Indicate the cranial nerve that innervates each extraocular muscle.

Muscle	Nerve
a. Lateral rectus	_____
b. Medial rectus	_____
c. Superior rectus	_____
d. Inferior rectus	_____
e. Superior oblique	_____
f. Inferior oblique	_____

3. In the position of primary gaze in the normal situation, the eyes are directed straight ahead and the visual axes of the two eyes are parallel. Keep in mind that in this position, all six extraocular muscles in each eye are tonically active and the position of the eye in the orbit reflects the combined, balanced actions of all six extraocular muscles contracting simultaneously. Any loss in the contractile force (weakness or paralysis) of a single extraocular muscle will result in movement of the eye about one or more axes produced by the relatively unopposed action of the remaining muscles. Indicate the effects on the eye resulting from paralysis of each of the extraocular muscles.

Muscle	Primary Effect	Secondary Effects	
a. Lateral rectus	_____		
b. Medial rectus	_____		
c. Superior rectus	_____	_____	_____
d. Inferior rectus	_____	_____	_____
e. Superior oblique	_____	_____	_____
f. Inferior oblique	_____	_____	_____

4. Extraocular muscle function can be evaluated by observing eye movement produced by each muscle when its action is exerted perpendicular to a single axis of rotation. Indicate the muscle being evaluated by each of the following movements.

a. Abduction of the eye   _____

b. Elevation of the abducted eye   _____

c. Depression of the abducted eye   _____

d. Adduction of the eye   _____

e. Elevation of the adducted eye   _____

f. Depression of the adducted eye   _____

5. Ocular malalignment (strabismus) can occur as a result of damage to the ocular motor nerves. Indicate the effects on the eye resulting from damage to each ocular motor nerve.

Nerve	**Resulting Eye Position**		
a. Abducens nerve	_____		
b. Trochlear nerve	_____	_____	_____
c. Oculomotor nerve	_____	_____	_____

6. Which cranial nerve, if damaged, will affect pupillary size? _____

   a. Will the pupil on the affected side be larger or smaller than the pupil on the uninvolved side? _____

7. Which cranial nerve, if damaged, will result in ptosis? _____

8. Which cranial nerve passes through the cavernous sinus, and as a result, can be damaged by intracavernous carotid artery aneurysms? _____

9. Which cranial nerve emerges from the dorsal surface of the brainstem?

   _____

Ear

INSPECTION

With the subject seated comfortably:

1. **Inspect the auricles, identifying the helix, antihelix, tragus, antitragus, and concha.**

    a. Are the right and left sides symmetrical? _____

    If not, describe the differences. _____

    _____

2. **Inspect the external acoustic meatus.**

3. **Using an otoscope, carefully examine the tympanic membrane.**

    a. In what direction does the "cone of light" extend from the umbo?

    _____

b. Which cranial nerves provide sensory innervation to the external surface of the tympanic membrane?

    1. _____

    2. _____

c. Which of the ossicles is attached to the internal surface of the tympanic membrane? _____

d. Which of the ossicles is attached to the oval window? _____

e. Which muscle attaches to the malleus? _____

    1. Which cranial nerve innervates this muscle? _____

f. Which muscle attaches to the stapes?_____

    1. Which cranial nerve innervates this muscle?_____

    2. Which cranial nerve transmits auditory impulses to the brainstem?

    _____

4. **Which foramen of the skull transmits the axons of the vestibulocochlear nerve?** _____

Answer Key

Section I. Limbs and Back

CHAPTER 1. SHOULDER GIRDLE AND UPPER LIMB

Inspection and Palpation

1. a.
   b.

2. a. gliding
   b. gliding

3. a.
   b.

4. a. acromion process
   b. T3
   c. supraspinatus
      1. suprascapular nerve
   d. infraspinatus
      1. suprascapular nerve

5. a. 5 cm
   b. 2nd
   c. 7th

6. a. pectoralis major
      1. medial and lateral pectoral nerves
   b. latissimus dorsi and teres major
      1. thoracodorsal nerve and lower subscapular nerve

7.　　a.　biceps brachii and brachialis
　　　　　　1.　musculocutaneous nerve
　　　b.

8.　　a.　triceps brachii
　　　　　　1.　radial nerve
　　　b.

9.　　a.　triceps brachii
　　　b.　ulnar nerve

10.　　a.　　1.　forearm pronation
　　　　　　　2.　wrist flexion
　　　　　　　3.　finger flexion

11.　　a.　　1.　forearm supination
　　　　　　　2.　wrist extension
　　　　　　　3.　finger extension

12.　　a.　pronator teres
　　　　　　1.　median nerve
　　　b.　brachioradialis
　　　　　　1.　radial nerve
　　　c.　brachial artery
　　　d.　median cubital vein
　　　e.　pronator teres
　　　f.　flexor carpi ulnaris

13.　　a.
　　　b.
　　　c.　radial nerve

14.　　a.
　　　b.
　　　c.　median nerve and ulnar nerve

15.　　a.
　　　b.
　　　c.
　　　d.　　1.　extensor pollicis longus

16.　　a.
　　　b.
　　　c.
　　　d.　radial artery
　　　e.　ulnar artery
　　　f.　median nerve

17.

18.　　a.
　　　b.　　1.　abductor pollicis brevis
　　　　　　　2.　flexor pollicis brevis
　　　　　　　3.　opponens pollicis
　　　c.　median nerve

       d.   1. abductor digiti minimi
              2. flexor digiti minimi
              3. opponens digiti minimi
       e. ulnar nerve

19.   a. extensor pollicis longus
       b.   1. abductor pollicis longus
              2. extensor pollicis brevis
       c. radial artery

20.   a.
       b. finger abduction
       c. ulnar nerve
       d. finger adduction
       e. ulnar nerve

Movement

1.	a.	trapezius	spinal accessory
		levator scapulae	dorsal scapular
2.	a.	rhomboid major	dorsal scapular
	b.	rhomboid minor	dorsal scapular
	c.	trapezius	spinal accessory
3.	a.	deltoid	axillary
4.	a.	deltoid	axillary
	b	supraspinatus	suprascapular
5.	a.	teres major	lower subscapular
	b.	teres minor	axillary
	c.	pectoralis major	pectoral (medial and lateral)
	d.	latissimus dorsi	thoracodorsal
6.	a.	deltoid	axillary
	b.	latissimus dorsi	thoracodorsal
7.	a.	biceps brachii	musculocutaneous
	b.	brachialis	musculocutaneous
8.	a.	brachioradialis	radial
	b.	brachialis	musculocutaneous
9.	a.	triceps brachii	radial
10.	a.	pronator teres	median
	b.	pronator quadratus	median
11.	a.	supinator	radial
	b.	biceps brachii	musculocutaneous
12.	a.	extensor carpi radialis longus	radial
	b.	extensor carpi radialis brevis	radial
	c.	extensor carpi ulnaris	radial
13.	a.	flexor carpi radialis	median
	b.	flexor carpi ulnaris	ulnar

14.	a. extensor carpi radialis longus	radial
	b. extensor carpi radialis brevis	radial
	c. flexor carpi radialis	median
15.	a. extensor carpi ulnaris	radial
	b. flexor carpi ulnaris	ulnar
16.	a. abductor pollicis longus	radial
	b. abductor pollicis brevis	median
17.	a. adductor pollicis	ulnar
18.	a. flexor pollicis longus	median
	b. flexor pollicis brevis	median
19.	a. extensor pollicis longus	radial
	b. extensor pollicis brevis	radial
	c. abductor pollicis longus	radial
20.	a. opponens pollicis	median
	b. opponens digiti minimi	ulnar
21.	a. lumbricales	median/ulnar
22.	a. extensor digitorum communis	radial
23.	a. dorsal interossei	ulnar
24.	a. palmar interossei	ulnar
25.	a. flexor digitorum superficialis	median
26.	a. flexor digitorum profundus	median/ulnar
27.	a. extensor digitorum communis	radial

Vasculature (Veins and Arteries)

1.

2.

Peripheral Nerves

1.

2.

3.

4.

5. a. anterior scalene
    b. middle scalene

Chapter 2. Hip Girdle and Lower Limb

Inspection and Palpation

1.

2. a. femoral artery
    b. femoral vein
    c. femoral nerve
    d.   1. sartorius
          2. adductor longus

3. a.
    b. rectus femoris
    c. anterior inferior iliac spine

4. a.
    b. prevents lateral displacement of the patella during knee extension

5. a. apex of patella
    b. tibial tubercle

6. a. common peroneal nerve
    b. soleus

7. a.   1. ankle dorsiflexion
          2. toe extension
    b. deep peroneal nerve
    c. anterior tibial artery

8. a.   1. peroneus longus
          2. peroneus brevis

9. a. plantar calcaneonavicular ligament

10. a.
    b.

11. a. anterior cruciate ligament
    b. anterior part of intercondylar eminence
    c. posteromedial surface of lateral femoral condyle

12. a. posterior cruciate ligament
    b. posterior part of intercondylar fossa
    c. anterolateral surface of medial femoral condyle

13. a. L4

14. a. sacrotuberous ligament
    b.   1. semitendinosus
          2. semimembranosus
          3. biceps femoris (long head)
          4. adductor magnus

15. a.
    b. knee flexion

16. a. biceps femoris
          1. tibial nerve (long head) and common peroneal nerve (short head)
    b. semitendinosus and semimembranosus
          1. tibial nerve
    c. gastrocnemius
          1. tibial nerve

    d. popliteal artery
    e. tibial nerve
    f. popliteus

17. a.
    b.   1. plantar flexion
          2. toe flexion
    c.   1. tibialis posterior
          2. flexor digitorum longus
          3. flexor hallucis longus

18. a.
    b. tibialis posterior

Movement

1.	a. psoas major	lumbar nerves
	b. iliacus	femoral
	c. rectus femoris	femoral
2.	a. quadriceps femoris	femoral
3.	a. tibialis anterior	deep peroneal
4.	a. gastrocnemius	tibial
	b. soleus	tibial
	c. tibialis posterior	tibial
5.	a. extensor hallucis longus	deep peroneal
	b. extensor digitorum longus	deep peroneal
	c. extensor digitorum brevis	deep peroneal
6.	a. flexor hallucis longus	tibial
	b. flexor digitorum longus	tibial
7.	a. gluteus maximus	inferior gluteal
8.	a. biceps femoris	tibial/common peroneal
	b. semitendinosus	tibial
	c. semimembranosus	tibial
9.	a. adductor magnus	obturator/tibial
	b. adductor longus	obturator
	c. adductor brevis	obturator
10.	a. gluteus medius	superior gluteal
	b. gluteus minimus	superior gluteal

Vasculature (Veins and Arteries)

1.

Nerves

1.

2.

3.

4.

Chapter 3. Back

Inspection and Palpation

1. a. there are curvatures in the sagittal plane
   b. 1. cervical
      2. lumbar
   c. lordosis
   d. 1. thoracic
      2. sacral
   e. kyphosis
   f. scoliosis

Movement

1. anterior longitudinal ligament

2. posterior longitudinal ligament

3. ligamentum flavum

4. intertransverse ligament

5. interspinous ligament

6. supraspinous

7. a. iliocostalis
   b. longissimus
   c. spinalis

8. a. semispinalis
   b. multifidus
   c. rotatores

9. a. splenius capitis
   b. splenius cervicis

10. a. obliquus capitis superior
    b. obliquus capitis inferior
    c. rectus capitis posterior major
    d. rectus capitis posterior minor

Section II. Thorax and Abdomen

Chapter 4. Thorax

Inspection and Palpation

1. a.

2. a. T2

3. a. T4
   b. 2nd rib

4. a. T9
    b. ribs 1-7
    c. ribs 8-10

5. a. ribs 11 and 12

6. a. posteriorly
    b. kyphosis

7. a.
    b.
    c.
    d.
    e. scoliosis

8.

9.

10. a. rib 2
    b. rib 7

Landmarks

1.

2.

3.

4. T4

CHAPTER 5. LUNGS AND PLEURA

Inspection and Palpation

1. a. expiration
    b. 12-18

2.

3.

Landmarks

1.

2. a. 8th rib
    b. 10th rib
    c. 12th rib

3. 6th costal cartilage

4. 4th costal cartilage

5.

6. a. 6th rib
    b. 8th rib
    c. 10th rib

7. 6th costal cartilage

8. 4th costal cartilage

9.

10. a. T3
    b. 5th
    c. 6th

11.

12. a. 5th rib
    b. 4th

13. a. 1. apical, posterior, anterior
       2. medial, lateral
       3. superior, anterior basal, lateral basal, posterior basal, medial basal
    b. 1. apico-posterior, anterior, superior (lingual), inferior (lingual)
       2. superior, anterior basal, lateral basal, posterior basal, medial basal

14. a. sternal angle
    b. T4 - T5 intervertebral disc

15. right

16. a. trapezius
    b. rhomboid major
    c. latissimus dorsi

17. 6th

18. a. T8
    b. T10
    c. T12

19. inferior vena cava

20. a. esophagus
    b. anterior and posterior vagal trunks

21. a. aorta
    b. azygos vein
    c. thoracic duct

CHAPTER 6. HEART

Landmarks

1. a.
   b.
   c.
   d.

2. a.
   b.
   c.
   d.

3. a.
   b.
   c.
   d.

Inspection and Palpation

1. a.

2. a.
   b.

Auscultation

1. a. S2
   b. S1
   c. S2
   d. S1

2. systole

CHAPTER 7. ABDOMEN

Inspection

1. a.
   b.
   c.

2. a.
   b.

3. a.
   b. above

Palpation and Landmarks

1.

2.

3.

4.

5.

6. a. L4

7. a. 1. liver
      2. gall bladder
      3. duodenum
      4. pancreas (head)
      5. right kidney
      6. hepatic flexure
   b. 1. stomach
      2. spleen

          3. pancreas (body)
          4. left kidney
          5. splenic flexure
    c. 1. appendix
          2. cecum
          3. right ovary
          4. right ureter
          5. ascending colon
    d. 1. left ovary
          2. left ureter
          3. descending colon
          4. sigmoid colon

8.

9.   a. L3
     b. 1. right hypochondriac
         2. epigastric
         3. left hypochondriac

10. a. L5
     b. 1. right lumbar
         2. umbilical
         3. left lumbar
     c. 1. right inguinal (iliac)
         2. hypogastric (pubic)
         3. left inguinal (iliac)

11. a. L4
     b. L1
     c. L5
     d. L3
     e. L2

12.

13. T10

14.

15.

Auscultation

1.   a. yes
     b.

Section III. Head and Neck

CHAPTER 8. HEAD AND FACE

Inspection and Palpation

1. a.
   b.

2. a. confluence of sinuses

3. a.
   b.
   c.
   d.
   e.
   f.   1. facial nerve

4. a.

5. a.

6. a.
   b. levator palpebrae superioris
       1. oculomotor nerve
   c.
   d.
   e.
   f.
   g.   1. orbicularis oculi
         2. facial nerve
   h.

7. a.

8. a.

9. a.

Movement

1.

2. a. trigeminal

3. a. frontalis
   b. facial nerve

4. a. orbicularis oculi
   b. facial nerve
   c. supraduction of the eye with forceful lid closure

5. a. risorius
   b. facial nerve

6. a. orbicularis oris
    b. facial nerve

7. internal auditory meatus

8. stylomastoid foramen

9. a. temporal
    b. zygomatic
    c. buccal
    d. mandibular
    e. cervical

Vasculature

1. a. external carotid artery

2.

3. a. external carotid artery

Peripheral Nerves

1. a. ophthalmic nerve
    b. maxillary nerve
    c. mandibular nerve

2. glossopharyngeal nerve
    a. otic ganglion

3. facial nerve
    a. submandibular ganglion

4. facial nerve
    a. pterygopalatine ganglion

5. facial nerve

6. trigeminal nerve

7. trigeminal nerve
    a. ophthalmic nerve
        1. superior orbital fissure
    b. maxillary nerve
        1. foramen rotundum
    c. mandibular nerve
        1. foramen ovale

8. jugular foramen

9. stylopharyngeus

10. a. blood pressure measurement by carotid sinus
     b. taste in posterior one-third of the tongue

11. jugular foramen

12. a. pharyngeal constrictors
     b. laryngeal muscles

13. slows heart rate

14. increases gastric and intestinal motility

15.   a. blood gas measurement by the carotid body
   b. taste on the epiglottis

16.   a. foramen magnum
   b. jugular foramen

17.   a. sternocleidomastoid
   b. trapezius

18. hypoglossal canal

19. genioglossus

CHAPTER 9. NECK

Inspection and Palpation

1.   a.
   b.

2.   a.   1. midline of neck
       2. anterior border of sternocleidomastoid
       3. inferior border of mandible
   b.   1. anterior border of sternocleidomastoid
       2. posterior belly of digastric
       3. superior belly of omohyoid
   c.   1. posterior belly of digastric
       2. anterior belly of digastric
       3. inferior border of mandible
   d.   1. superior belly of omohyoid
       2. anterior border of sternocleidomastoid
       3. midline of neck
   e.   1. sternohyoid
       2. sternothyroid
       3. thyrohyoid

3.

4.   a. C3
   b.   1. digastric
       2. stylohyoid
       3. mylohyoid
       4. geniohyoid

5.   a. C5

6.   a. up
   b. posterior cricoarytenoid
   c. inferior laryngeal
   d.   1. lateral cricoarytenoid
       2. transverse arytenoid
   e. inferior laryngeal

      f. cricothyroid
      g. external laryngeal
      h. internal laryngeal

7.   a. C6

8.   a.   1. sternothyroid
         2. thyrohyoid
         3. sternohyoid
         4. omohyoid

9.   a.

10.   a. C7

11.   a.   1. anterior border of trapezius
         2. posterior border of sternocleidomastoid
         3. superior border of clavicle
    b.
    c.   1. splenius capitis
         2. levator scapulae
         3. scalenus posterior
         4. scalenus medius
    d. rotation to the contralateral side

12.   a.

Vasculature

1.   a. C4

2.   a. vagus nerve
    b. internal jugular vein

3.   a. carotid tubercle
    b.

CHAPTER 10. MOUTH

Inspection and Palpation

1.   a.

2.   a. masseter
    b. trigeminal

3.   a.

4.   a.
    b. glossopharyngeal
    c. palatoglossus
    d. palatopharyngeus

5.   a.

Movements

1. a.
    b. levator veli palatini
    c. vagus

2. a.
    b. genioglossus
    c. hypoglossal
    d. trigeminal
    e. facial

CHAPTER 11. EYE

Inspection

1. a.
    b.

2. a.
    b.
    c.
    d.

3.

4. a. anisocoria

5. a. pupillary constriction
    b. pupillary constriction
    c. direct light reflex
    d. indirect (consensual) light reflex

6. a. pupillary constriction
    b. pupillary constriction

7. a.
    b. strabismus
    c.
    d. nystagmus

Movements

1. a. abduction
    b. adduction
    c. supraduction   intorsion   adduction
    d. subduction   extorsion   adduction
    e. intorsion   subduction   abduction
    f. extorsion   supraduction   abduction

2. a. abducens
    b. oculomotor
    c. oculomotor
    d. oculomotor
    e. trochlear
    f. oculomotor

3. a. adducted
    b. abducted

c. subducted	extorted	abducted
d. supraducted	intorted	abducted
e. extorted	supraducted	adducted
f. intorted	subducted	adducted

4. a. lateral rectus
    b. superior rectus
    c. inferior rectus
    d. medial rectus
    e. inferior oblique
    f. superior oblique

5. a. adducted

b. extorted	supraducted	adducted
c. subducted	abducted	intorted

6. oculomotor
    a. larger

7. oculomotor

8. abducens

9. trochlear

Chapter 12. Ear

Inspection

1. a

2.

3. a. anteriorly and inferiorly
    b.   1. trigeminal
         2. vagus
    c. malleus
    d. stapes
    e. tensor tympani
         1. trigeminal
    f. stapedius
         1. facial
         2. cochlear nerve

4. internal auditory meatus

INDEX